Fatty Liver Cookbook

Nutritional Diet Plan To Eliminate Toxic, Lose Stubborn Fat And Reverse Liver Disease

Sara Williams

Copyright © 2018 Sara Williams

All rights reserved. No part of this publication may be reproduced, distributed, or transmitted in any form or by any means, including photocopying, recording, or other electronic or mechanical methods, without the prior written permission of the publisher, except in the case of brief quotations embodied in critical reviews and certain other noncommercial uses permitted by copyright law.

Limit of Liability

The information in this book is solely for informational purposes, not as a medical instruction to replace the advice of your physician or as a replacement for any treatment prescribed by your physician. The author and publisher do not take responsibility for any possible consequences from any treatment, procedure, exercise, dietary modification, action or application of medication which results from reading or following the information contained in this book.

If you are ill or suspect that you have a medical problem, we strongly encourage you to consult your medical, health, or other competent professional before adopting any of the suggestions in this book or drawing inferences from it.

This book and the author's opinions are solely for informational and educational purposes. The author specifically disclaims all responsibility for any liability, loss, or risk, personal or otherwise

All rights reserved. No part of this publication may be reproduced, distributed or transmitted in any form or by any means, including photocopying, Recording, or other electronic or mechanical methods, without the prior written Permission of the publisher, except in the case of brief quotations embodied in Critical reviews and certain other noncommercial uses permitted by copyright Law.

ISBN: 9781687115102

TABLE OF CONTENT

INTRODUCTION

Understanding Your Liver

What Are The Known Symptoms Of Fatty Liver?

   Types of fatty liver disease

Who Is At Potential Risk Of Having Fatty Liver?

Ways To diagnose a Fatty Liver?

Tips And Strategies On How To Reverse And Treat Fatty Liver.

Natural Foods That Can Help You Reverse Fatty Liver

   Tips On How To Cook With Less Fat

FATTY LIVER RECIPES

DRINKS

   Healthy Vacation Peach Drink

   Easy Pumpkin Spice Latte

   Pineapple, Watermelon Smoothie

   Ginger Honey Lemonade

   Perfect "Shamrock" Shake

   Green Pumpkin Spice Smoothie

   Summer Oat Berry Smoothie

   Sweet Berry Banana Yogurt Smoothie

   Banana Apple Smoothie

   Eastertide Nectarine Smoothie

BREAKFAST RECIPES

   Sunrise Apple With Bananas Oats Milkshake

   Liver Cure Breakfast Granola

   Banana Blueberry Pancakes

   Walnuts Almond Milk Apple Oats

   Easy Chilled Garlic Hummus

   Homemade Roasted seeds, Gluten Free, Nut Free recipe

- Breakfast Toasted Bread With Cheese Omelet
- Chia Seed honey Yogurt Custard
- Granny's Healthy Oatmeal
- Steel Cut Oats with Strawberries and Almond

LUNCH RECIPES

- Portobello Oregano "Philly Cheese Steak Wheat Rolls
- Organic Black Bean Oat Brownies
- Scallion, Green Onion Mushroom Omelet
- Tossed Mango Salsa With Local Bean
- Goody Choco Rice Krispies
- Fresh Turmeric Brown Rice
- Oven Roasted Bok Choy
- Turkey Veggie Stuffed Peppers
- Broccoli Avocado Cucumber Salad
- Ocean Breeze Edamame Toss
- Leftover Chicken Anchor Grape Salad
- Roasted Vegetable Broccoli Pesto Bowls
- Chicken Sausage & Red Onion Pasta
- Greek-Way Oregano Chicken Salad

DINNER RECIPES

- Potato Basil Chickpea Cacciatore
- Whole-Wheat Spaghetti Lemon with Salmon
- Mixed Vegetable Meal
- Baked Chilli Lime Chicken
- Garlic Cilantro Lime Rice
- Coconut Zucchinis Curry Fish
- Sweet Potato With Kale Chili Portobello
- Sweet Potato With Lentil Bolognese Noodles
- Turkey Meatloaf With Tomato Ketchup

Merry Spanakopita

Zucchinis Mushrooms, Fettuccini Alfredo

DESSERTS RECIPES

Vanilla Cashew Bites

Oats With Peanut Butter Granola Bars

Quick Starter Lime Mousse

Yankee Spicy Stewed Apples

Quick Cheese Prosciutto Peaches

Plum Nut Almond Crumble Muffin

Mango Vanilla Tiramisù

Orange Cherry Crisp

Pineapple Mango Lemon Cream

Pecan Peanut Butter Banana Cake

SALADS RECIPES

Beets Steamed Edamame Salad

Avocado Cilantro Chunky Salsa

Potatoes Mixed Vegetables

Toasted Mango Pepitas Kale Salad

Chickpea And Parsley Pumpkin Salad

White Bean Cherry Tomatoes Cucumber Salad

Arugula Cucumber Tuna Salad

Springtime Chicken Berries Salad

Toaster Almond Spiralized Beet Salad

SOUPS RECIPES

Apple Leeks Mascarpone Soup

Aminos Mushroom Soup

Detox-Liver Arugula And Broccoli Soup

Pasta Veggies Minestrone Soup

Unique Lentil with Kale Soup

Pear Red Pepper Soup

Low Heat Chicken Provençal

Danny's Tortellini Soup

Wellness Parsnip Soup

Feel Good Chicken Soup

SNACKS RECIPES

Boneless Chicken Guacamole

Easy Fresh Guacamole

Garlic Chili Pita Chips

Hearty Masala Lotus Seed

Roasted Spiced Chickpeas Crispy

Honey Nut Raisins Granola

Cornmeal Cauliflower Fritters

Vanilla Chocolate Macaroon Bars

Tasty Peach Crumble

Grilled Veggies With Tofu Skewers

INTRODUCTION

Understanding Your Liver

Fatty liver is also known as "hepatic steatosis", a condition associated with having too many fat deposits in the liver. Although it is not unusual to see a few traces of fat present in the liver, having it in excess can result in a health issue. It only becomes an issue when the liver is overloaded with so much fat that it hinders it from functioning optimally, which can pose a real health danger. The liver, being the largest internal organ in the body, helps with the proper processing of nutrients from food and drinks, and filters the blood of many harmful substances.

The liver also performs these among many functions:
Enzyme activation
Production of bile and excretion
Excretion of hormones, bilirubin, cholesterol and drugs
Metabolism of carbohydrates, fats, and proteins
It helps to synthesize plasma proteins.
Blood purification and detoxification
It stores glycogen, minerals and vitamins.

What Are The Known Symptoms Of Fatty Liver?

I will say the unfortunate thing about this disease is that most people living with the condition do not know that they have it, and sadly, there is a great danger if left untreated.

Mostly, fatty liver causes no apparent symptoms but anyone with fatty liver condition may feel tired easily or experience constant pain or discomfort in the right side of the upper abdomen. Sometimes, it may lead to more server condition such as liver scarring. Another name for liver scarring is liver fibrosis. A severe liver fibrosis condition is known as cirrhosis.

Cirrhosis may cause symptoms like:
Yellow skin and eyes
Confusion
Breast enlargement in men
Swelling of your legs
Abdominal swelling
Abdominal pain
Web-like clusters of blood vessels under your skin

Itchy skin
Nosebleeds
Fatigue
Weakness
Weight loss
Loss of appetite

Types of fatty liver disease

Fatty liver is divided into two types:
1) Alcoholic fatty liver disease, also called alcoholic steatohepatitis.
2) Nonalcoholic fatty liver disease (NAFLD).

1) Alcoholic fatty liver disease:
Alcoholic steatohepatitis occurs because of excessive alcoholic drinking. Drinking excessively can damage the liver, and the liver will not be able to perform the function of breaking down fat properly. Alcoholic fatty liver is the first stage of ARLD which rarely causes any symptoms, but it's a bad signal that your drinking rate can be very harmful.
If there are no other complications or inflammation along with the build-up of fat around the liver, it is known as simple alcoholic fatty liver.
Alcoholic steatohepatitis (ASH)
ASH is a liver condition accompanied by inflammation. If not treated properly, it can lead to a higher chance of liver cancer, liver failure, alcoholic hepatitis, or cirrhosis.

2) Nonalcoholic Fatty Liver Disease:

Nonalcoholic Fatty Liver Disease is becoming the most common type of fatty liver disease, largely due to poor diets. Patients with suspected or confirmed diagnosis are advised to follow nutritional recommendations, which is a kind of healthy diet where you have to switch from the consumption of mainly refined grains to whole grains. Even after following a healthy fatty liver diet, there is also a need for an increase in physical activity to promote weight loss.

Nonalcoholic Fatty Liver Disease is usually not harmful, but the condition can develop into an advanced stage called (NASH) Nonalcoholic steatohepatitis. When the liver condition is accompanied with inflammation without any trace of alcohol, your doctor may diagnose you with NASH.
At this stage, the liver becomes swollen and can also result in a scare in your liver that won't heal (cirrhosis).

This can open door to issues like:
Heart disease or a chance of liver cancer
Drowsiness, confusion, and slurred speech (hepatic encephalopathy)
Ascites: fluid buildup in the abdomen
Esophageal varices: This is the swelling of veins in the esophagus.
Liver failure occurs when your liver finally stops functioning.

Some Symptoms of Fatty Liver
Fatty liver causes no apparent symptoms, but at some point, some people might experience various symptoms like:
Abdominal pain
Loss of appetite
Become very tired
Excessive weight loss and nausea

Who Is At Potential Risk Of Having Fatty Liver?

People with a higher risk of developing fatty liver disease are obese or overweight; people with high blood pressure, people with type 2 diabetes, triglycerides and high cholesterol, or other liver infections.

Other factors that add to the risk of fatty liver:
Malnutrition
Underactive pituitary gland (hypopituitarism)
High cholesterol
Absent of good physical activity
Pregnancy
Metabolic syndrome
High triglyceride levels
Underactive thyroid (hypothyroidism)
Metabolic syndrome
Overuse of some certain medications, like acetaminophen (Tylenol)
Excessive consumption of alcohol

Ways To diagnose Fatty Liver

1) Ultrasound and other types of imaging studies. Using an ultrasound can help to detect if you have fat in your liver. More so, other imaging studies can be done as well, such as MRI or CT scans.

2) Fibro Scan

Similar to ultra sound, it makes use of sound waves to determine the normal liver tissue, density of the liver and correlating areas of fat.

3) Fatty liver can also be detected by your doctor after inspecting your abdomen for an enlarged liver. Checks like this may not be 100% accurate, so it is your responsibility to explain to your doctor what kind of symptoms you are experiencing, as well as any medication, supplement, or alcohol use.

4) Liver biopsy
Many experts refer to this as the most effective way to detect the severity of liver disease and also the exact cause. It is done by inserting a needle into the liver to extract a piece of tissue; the tissue is then examined to detect a liver disease. A local anesthetic will be given to reduce the pain.

5) Blood tests
If there is an unusual increase in the liver enzymes during a routine blood test, this can be related to liver inflammation but does not ascertain a fatty liver disease. Running a blood test may help to discover the risk of fatty liver, although further analysis should be carried out.

Tips And Strategies, On How To Reverse And Treat Fatty Liver Disease.

The easiest way to reverse and treat fatty liver disease is by eating a well-balanced diet.
Remove or reduce fatty foods and foods that have a high level of sugar from your diet, such as duck, pork belly, fried chips, crisps, nuts etc.
Eat lots of veggies.
Avoid red meat.
Avoid eating processed foods; most of them have high fat content, like lasagna, pizza, etc.
It is best to eat lean proteins such as fish, turkey, chicken, and soy, whole grains, and good-for-you fats.
Sodas, juices and any sweet drink should be eliminated.
Substitute high fat margarine, butter, lard, dripping, and mayonnaise with low-fat substitutes.
Substitute full cream milk with skimmed or semi-skimmed milk.
You can reverse fatty liver automatically when the necessary steps are taken to treat obesity, an unhealthy diet, diabetes, and high cholesterol.

Exercise regularly; it helps you get rid of excess liver fat. Small workouts, brisk walking, etc.

Stop drinking alcohol. This might not be easy for some people, but it's something you need to work on for your overall health benefit.

Reduce carbs and sugar intake

Be kind to your liver, mindful of your medications, especially the ones that can cause fatty liver.

Natural Foods That Can Help You Reverse Fatty Liver

Fish for inflammation and fat levels
Fish such as trout, tuna, sardines, and salmon have high level of omega-3 fatty acids which can assist in bringing down inflammation and improve liver fat levels.

Sunflower seeds as antioxidants
Vitamin E is a high-antioxidant that helps protect the liver from damage. Sunflower seeds are rich in vitamin E.

Garlic
Apart from adding flavor to food, it also helps reduce fat and body weight in people with fatty liver disease.

Milk and other low-fat dairy
Milk and other low-fat dairy may assist to protect the liver from more damage because of the presence of whey protein.

Walnuts
Walnuts are high in omega-3 fatty acids, which help to improve the liver.

Fruits
Especially citrus fruits, it has essential vitamins that are beneficial for health with great potential for fatty liver treatment.

Coffee helps to reduce abnormal liver enzymes.
Research has revealed that people who love to drink coffee have a lower risk of liver damage. Caffeine helps to reduce abnormal liver enzymes and the risk of liver diseases.

Olive oil for weight control

Olive oil contains a high concentration of omega-3 fatty acids, which can help lower liver enzyme levels, reduce inflammation, and improve liver fat levels.

Oatmeal
Oatmeal has fiber content that can help weight maintenance. More so, the carbohydrates present in whole grains like oatmeal is a good source of body energy.

Avocados help protect the liver.
Fruits like avocados and nuts. Avocados contain chemicals that have the ability to slow liver damage and are also rich in healthy fats.

Greens prevent fat buildup.

Eat enough greens like kale, spinach, Brussels sprouts, and spinach. It helps to reduce weight. Spinach helps to prevent fat building up in the liver.

Green tea for less fat absorption.

Green tea improves liver function and storage in the liver. Green tea is also beneficial in many ways, aiding with sleep and lowering cholesterol.

Tofu to reduce fat buildup

FATTY LIVER RECIPES

DRINKS

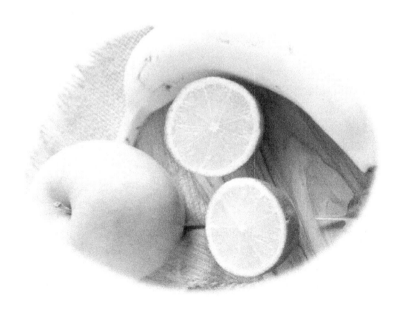

Healthy Vacation Peach Drink

Prep time: 5 minutes
Cook time: 5 minutes
Servings: 4-5

Ingredients:
2 fresh lemon juice
Ice cubes
10 tbsp of sweetener of choice
5 cups of water
8 peeled peaches, cut into slices
For garnish:
Mint leaves
Peach slices

Instructions:
1. Add peach slices, sweetener of choice, lemon juice, ice cubes and water in the bowl of your blender and blend on medium speed. Blend again until smooth.
2. Pour peach drink over ice in a glass and garnish with mint leaves and peach slice, if desired.

Easy Pumpkin Spice Latte

Prep time: 5 minutes
Cook time: 5 minutes
Servings: 2

Ingredients:
1 tsp of vanilla, alcohol-free
Pinch of cinnamon
16 ounces of fresh-brewed coffee
4-6 drops of liquid stevia
1 cup of vanilla almond milk, unsweetened
2 tsp of pumpkin pie spice
6 tbsp of pumpkin puree

Instructions:
1. Combine pumpkin and almond milk together in a saucepan, and cook over medium heat until hot (not boiling) or place in the microwave for 30 to 45 seconds.
2. Stir in spices, vanilla, and sweetener.
3. Transfer the mix to a blender and blend until foamy, about 30 seconds.
4. Add the milk mixture into coffee, and top with cinnamon.

Pineapple, Watermelon Smoothie

Prep time: 5 minutes
Cook time: 5 minutes
Servings: 6

Ingredients:
1 1/2 cups of coconut milk.
2 1/2 teaspoons of honey (optional)
5 teaspoons of freshly grated turmeric.
5 cups of cubed frozen watermelon
3 1/2 cups of cubed frozen coconut water
1 1/2 orange, peeled, seeds removed
5 cups of fresh cubed frozen pineapple
2 1/2 teaspoons of fresh ginger, grated

Instructions:
1. Add together all the ingredients in the bowl of your blender and blend until a smooth mixture emerges.
2. Add honey if using, blend, and serve.

Ginger Honey Lemonade

Prep time: 2 minutes
Cook time: 13 minutes
Servings: 4

Ingredients:
Lemon slices for garnish, if desired
1 medium sprigs of fresh rosemary
Ice cubes
1/6 cup of honey
1/2 large sprig of fresh rosemary for garnish, if desired
2 large strips of lemon peel
1 tbsp of fresh ginger root, grated
Juice of 2 lemons

Instructions:
1. Combine together sprigs of fresh rosemary, lemon peel, ginger, honey and add 1 cup of water to a small pot.
3. Let cool about 15 minutes then strain mixture into large pitcher. Discard the rosemary and ginger.
4. Add in the 2 lemon juice and three cups of cold water to pitcher, mix to combine.
5. To serve, pour over ice along with lemon slice and little piece of fresh rosemary as garnish, if desired.

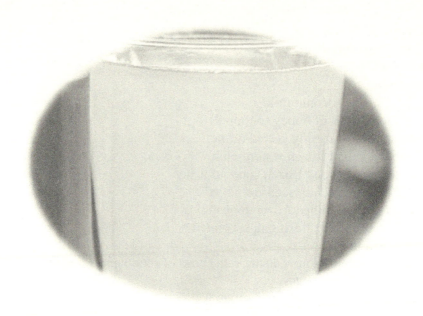

Perfect "Shamrock" Shake

Prep time: 2 minutes
Cook time: 3 minutes
Servings: 4
Ingredients:
2 scoop of Ultra Nourish
1 teaspoon of mint extract, alcohol-free
3 cups of vanilla almond milk
4 cups of vanilla frozen yogurt
Instructions:
1. Combine every ingredient in a blender and blend to have a smooth mixture. Enjoy!

Green Pumpkin Spice Smoothie

Prep time: 4 minutes
Cook time: 2 minutes
Servings: 2
Ingredients:
1/2 teaspoon of ground ginger
Pinch of ground nutmeg
2 handfuls of ice cubes
Pinch of ground cloves

2 cup sweetened, vanilla almond milk
Pinch of allspice
1/2 teaspoon of ground cinnamon
2 tablespoon honey
1 cup of canned pumpkin
1 ripe banana, peeled
2 scoop of Ultra Nourish (PROTEIN POWDER)

Instructions:
1. Combine together the entire ingredients in a blender and blend to have a smooth mixture.
2. Adjust spice and sweetness to taste, serve and enjoy!

Summer OatBerry Smoothie

Prep time: 4 minutes
Cook time: 3 minutes
Servings: 3

Ingredients:
3 cups of almond milk
3 cups of mixed frozen berries (blackberries, blueberries, raspberries, strawberries)
3 tbsp of your preferred nut butter
3/4 cup of oats
3 scoop of Ultra Nourish

Instructions:
1. Pour the oats in the bowl of your food processor and process to make a powder.
2. Pour in the rest ingredients and blend until you have a smooth mixture. Serve and enjoy.

Sweet Berry Banana Yogurt Smoothie

Prep time: 2 minutes
Cook time: 5 minutes
Servings: 3

Ingredients:
3 (15 ounces) container of Greek yogurt
3 scoop of Ultra Nourish
3 cups of unsweetened juice of your choice
3 bananas cut into small sizes
3/4 cup of blueberries
Several strawberries, halved
1 cup crushed ice

Instructions:
1. Combine together the entire ingredients in a blender and blend until you have a smooth mixture. Enjoy!

Banana Apple Smoothie

Prep time: 5 minutes
Cook time: 5 minutes
Servings: 4

Instructions:
2 cup (8 oz.) almond milk
2 tbsp of almond butter or natural peanut butter
2 scoop Ultra Nourish
1 frozen banana, cut into small sizes
2 cored and sliced apple

Instructions:
1. Whisk together the entire ingredients in a blender and blend until you have a smooth mixture.
Note: frozen bananas will make the texture thicker and won't require ice to chill the smoothie.

Eastertide Nectarine Smoothie

Prep time: 5 minutes
Cook time: 5 minutes
Servings: 2

Ingredients:
4 tbsp of whey protein powder
2 tbsp of ground flaxseeds
3 cups of water
4 tbsp of canned coconut cream
2 large nectarines

Instructions:
1. Combine the entire ingredients in a blender and blend until you have a smooth mixture.

BREAKFAST RECIPES

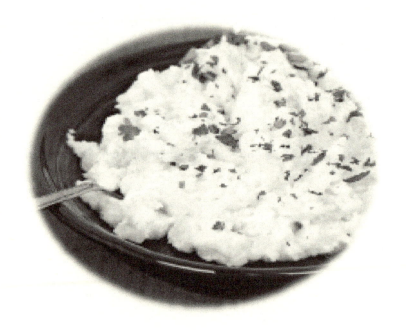

Sunrise Apple With Bananas Oats Milkshake

Prep time: 5 minutes
Cook time: 5 minutes
Servings: 2

Ingredients:
1/2 tbsp of chopped almonds
1/2 cup of quick cooking rolled oats
1/2 tbsp of chopped walnuts
1 1/2 cups of reduced-fat milk, 99.7% fat-free, chilled
1 1/2 tbsp of raisins
1 1/2 tsp sweetener
1/2 cup of apples, chopped (unpeeled)
1/2 cup of sliced bananas
1/8 tsp of vanilla essence

Instructions:
1. Combine together the chopped almonds, oats and chopped walnuts in a non-stick fry-pan, lightly roast over low heat for 4 to 5 minutes, stirring constantly. Set aside to cool completely.
2. Add the raisins and vanilla essence and stir well. Keep secure in an airtight container.
3. Pour the oat/nut mixture, chopped apples, sliced bananas and sweetener into a bowl. Pour the reduced-fat milk over it and stir well. Serve immediately.

Liver Cure Breakfast Granola

Prep time: 3 minutes
Cook time: 35-40 minutes
Servings: 5-6

Ingredients:
1 1/2 teaspoon of cinnamon
3 cup of dried cranberries, or preferred dried chopped fruit
1 cup of good honey
1 cup of applesauce
12 cups of organic rolled oats (it's different from quick cooking oats)
1 cup of apple cider or apple juice
1 teaspoon of salt or more
6 tbsp of flax seeds
5 tbsp of brown sugar

3 cup of shredded coconut
1 1/2 cup of hazelnuts, chopped
1 1/2 cup of almonds, chopped
3/4 teaspoon of nutmeg

Instructions:
1. Turn up the oven to 300 degrees F. Lined parchment paper over a large sheet pan.
2. Whisk together the flax seeds, oats, nutmeg, cinnamon, coconut, brown sugar, nuts, and salt in a large mixing bowl.
3. Whisk together the apple juice, honey, and applesauce in a different bowl.
4. Combine the wet mixture with the dry mixture and stir until you have a well-combined mixture.
5. Spread the granola evenly onto the prepared pan.
6. Bake in the oven and keep stirring once in 10 minutes, until the mixture turns golden brown and nice, about 30 to 40 minutes.
7. Withdraw from the oven and let the granola cool completely, stirring once a bit. Stir in the cranberries. Top granola with almond milk or yogurt. It can be stored in a plastic bag or an airtight container and refrigerated for weeks.

Banana Blueberry Pancakes

Prep time: 5 minutes
Cook time: 5 minutes
Servings: 2-4

Ingredients:
1 cup of fresh blueberries
1/4 tsp of baking powder
Butter and maple syrup for serving, (if desired.
4 large eggs at room temperature
3 ripe bananas, peeled

Instructions:
1. Mash the 3 ripe bananas in a mixing bowl using a potato masher or a fork, leaving it slightly lumpy.
2. Crack the eggs open and whisk in a separate bowl.
3. Combine together the eggs and mashed bananas, then mix in the baking powder. Mix thoroughly until well incorporated. Set aside
4. Meanwhile, heat a sauté pan over medium heat.
5. Coat the sauté pan with cooking spray, add four tbsp batter onto the hot sauté pan.

6. Place a small amount of blueberries into the batter. When the top of the pancake begins to produce small bubbles, flip the pancake and cook the other side. Serve warm with a dollop of butter and/or maple syrup on top.

Walnuts Almond Milk Apple Oats

Prep time: 5 minutes
Cook time: 3 minutes
Servings: 4
Ingredients:
1 cup of quick cooking rolled oats
3 tablespoon of dates, finely chopped
1/2 cup of apple, chopped (unpeeled)
2 cups of readymade almond milk
2 tablespoons of walnuts, chopped
1/2 tsp of cinnamon powder
Instructions:
1. Combine together all the ingredient (with the exception of walnuts and apples) in a large non-stick pan over medium heat.
2. Cook for about 2 to 3 minutes, stirring occasionally until heated through.
3. Add the walnuts and apples and mix thoroughly. Serve immediately.

Easy Chilled Garlic Hummus

Prep time: 15 minutes
Cook time: 0 minutes
Servings: 3
Ingredients:
3 tablespoons of red chili paste
3/4 teaspoon of olive oil, for drizzling
4 tablespoons of olive oil
3 cup of white chick peas (soaked and boiled)
1 1/2 tablespoon of garlic, roughly chopped
3/4 cup of curds
6 tbsp of water
Salt to taste
Instructions:

1. Add the entire ingredients together in a mixer and blend until a smooth mixture emerges.

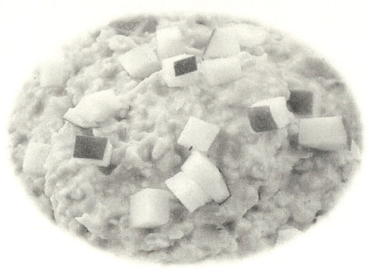

Homemade Roasted seeds, Gluten Free, Nut Free recipe
Prep time: 5 minutes
Cook time: 18 minutes
Servings: 2 1/2 cups
Ingredients:
1/2 cup of raw sunflower seeds
1/2 cup of chia seeds
1/2 cup of flax seeds
1/2 cup of raw pumpkin seeds
1/2 cup of hemp seeds
Instructions:
1. Place the hemp seeds in a non-stick pan, dry roast the hemp seeds in the pan over medium heat for about 4 to 5 minutes, tossing occasionally. Set aside in a bowl.
2. Place the pumpkin seeds and dry roast on medium heat inside the same pan for 4 minutes, tossing occasionally. Set aside in a bowl.
3. Place the sunflower seeds, dry roast sunflower seeds in the same pan on medium heat for 3 minutes, tossing occasionally. Set aside to cool completely.
4. Add chai seed and flax seed, then repeat step 3.
5. Pour hemp seeds into a mixer and blend until they become a smooth powder. Set aside
6. Add, chia seeds, flax seeds, sunflower seeds, and pumpkin seeds, then repeat step.
7. In a deep bowl, add smooth powders and mix to combine.
8. Store in the refrigerator in an air-tight container and use as required.

Breakfast Toasted Bread With Cheese Omelet

Prep time: 10 minutes
Cook time: 6 minutes
Servings: 4

Ingredients:
6 eggs
1 teaspoon of dried mixed herbs
2 teaspoons of green chilies, finely chopped
Salt and black pepper, freshly ground to taste
4 teaspoons of butter
1/2 cup of tomatoes, deseeded and chopped finely
1/2 cup of grated cheese, processed
1/2 cup capsicum, finely chopped
1/2 cup of onions, finely chopped
For Serving
Toasted bread slices and tomato ketchup

Instructions:
1. In a deep mixing bowl, whisk together 6 eggs, pepper, and salt.
2. Combine together the chopped capsicm, freshly ground black pepper, onions, tomatoes and green chilies with the exception of butter, and mix very well.
3. In a large non-stick pan over medium heat, melt the butter and pour in the egg mixture. Cook for 2 minutes.
4. Flip to cook the other side for 2 minutes more.
5. Place cheese beside the omelet and sprinkle evenly with dried mixed herbs.
6. Fold the omelet into half and cook for 60 seconds over medium heat. Serve with toasted bread slices and tomato ketchup on the side.

Chia Seed honey Yogurt Custard

Prep time: 10 minutes
Cook time: 10 minutes
Servings: 4 cups

Ingredients:
1/2 cup of freshly squeezed orange juice
12 tbsp of chia seeds
1 tsp of cinnamon
4 tbsp of honey
1 tsp of ground sumac
1 tsp of vanilla extract
2 cup of kefir yogurt or plain live
1 1/2 cups of coconut milk

Instructions:
1. Combine together the sumac, cinnamon and chia seeds in a blender and blend just enough to form a coarse powder.
2. Add in the honey, milk, yogurt, vanilla and orange juice. Blend about four or five times, the consistency of the mixture should resemble a thick soup.
3. Let it sit for about an hour or overnight in the fridge to form a thicker, custard like mix.

Granny's Healthy Oatmeal

Prep time: 10 minutes
Cook time: 8 minutes
Servings: 4

Ingredients:
1 cup of raisins (organic, if possible)
2 cup of water
2 teaspoon of clover honey
1 cup of steel rolled oats
2 teaspoon of pure maple syrup
2 teaspoon of ground cinnamon

Instructions:
1. Bring water to a boil in a pan and cook the steel-rolled oats according to manufacturer directions. You can add salt if you want. Add the raisins, maple syrup, honey and ground cinnamon. Stir thoroughly.

Steel Cut Oats with Strawberries and Almond

Prep time: 10 minutes
Cook time 8 minutes
Servings: 4

Ingredients:
1 cup of almond milk
2 tbsp of roasted almond halves
4 tsp of maple syrup
1 1/2 cup of strawberry cubes
1 cup of steel cut oats, soaked in water for 8 hours, drained
1/2 tsp of vanilla essence
2 cups of water

Instructions:
1. Bring 2 cups of water to a boil in a non-stick pan, add oats and mix well.
2. Cook with the lid on, over a medium low heat for 6 minutes, stirring not too often. Set the mixture aside to cool in a large bowl.
3. Add the maple syrup, 1 cup of strawberries, vanilla essence, and almond milk, and stir well.
4. Top with roasted almonds and the reserved 1/2 cup of strawberries. Serve right away or store it in the fridge.

LUNCH RECIPES

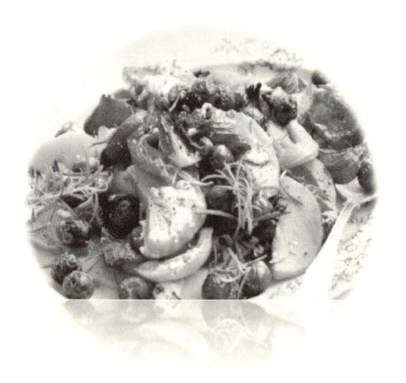

Portobello Oregano "Philly Cheese Steak Wheat Rolls

Prep time: 5 minutes.
Cook time: 15 minutes
Servings: 2

Ingredients:

1/4 tsp of freshly ground pepper
2 split and toasted, whole-wheat rolls
1/2 tbsp of all-purpose flour
1.5 Oz of reduced-fat provolone cheese, thinly sliced
1/8 cup of vegetable broth
1/2 tbsp of reduced-sodium soy sauce
1 tsp of dried oregano
1 tsp of extra-virgin olive oil
1/2 large red bell pepper, thinly sliced
2 large sliced Portobello mushrooms, gills and stems removed
1/2 sliced medium onion

Instructions:

1. In a broad nonstick pan, sauté the diced onions in olive oil over medium-high heat. Cook for about 5 minutes, stirring frequently, until tender and starting to brown.
2. Add in the dried oregano, freshly ground pepper, mushrooms and bell pepper.
3. Cook about 7 minutes, stirring frequently until the vegetables are tender.
4. Lower the heat and sprinkle half tablespoon of all-purpose flour on the vegetables. Stir to coat. Stir in soy sauce and broth; bring to a simmer.
5. Turn off heat and place slices of the provolone cheese on the vegetables, cover with a lid and let stand for 1 to 2 minutes until cheese melts on top.
6. Spoon the mixture with a spatula into two serving portions, keeping the melted cheese layer on top. Serve immediately by Spooning a portion of the mixture onto each toasted whole-wheat rolls.

Organic Black Bean Oat Brownies

Prep time: 20 minutes
Cook time: 18 minutes
Servings: 4-6

Ingredients:
1/4 cup of pure maple syrup
1/4 cup of chocolate chips
1 tsp of pure vanilla extract, alcohol-free
1/8 tsp of salt
1/8 cup of coconut oil
1/2 7-oz can of organic black beans, drained and rinsed
1/4 cup of quick oats
1 tbsp of cocoa powder
1/4 tsp of baking powder

Instructions:
1. Heat up your oven to 350 F.
2. Add the entire ingredients into the bowl of your food processor, but reserve the chips; Process until fully incorporated and smooth. Add the chocolate chips, stir.
3. Transfer the mixture into the oven and bake it for about 18 minutes.
4. Allow cooling completely out of the oven before cutting. Texture might look too soft. If not satisfied with the texture, chill in the refrigerator overnight to firm up.

Scallion, Green Onion Mushroom Omelet

Prep time: 3 minutes
Cook time: 5 minutes
Servings: 3

Ingredients:
3 tsp of minced garlic
3/4 cup of chopped kale
3/4 cup of chopped green onion
3 tbsp of low fat sour cream or heavy cream
3/4 cup of diced tomato
6 eggs
Optional additions:
3/4 cup of diced mushroom
3 scoops of Daily Turmeric Tonic
3/8 cup of diced Serrano pepper
3/4 cup of chopped bell pepper

Instructions:
1. Beat the sour cream and eggs together in a mixing bowl until smooth and fluffy.
2. Sauté the onion, kale, tomato, and garlic for 2-3 minutes in oil in a small non-stick pan over medium heat until soft. Add optional ingredients if using any.
3. Add in the beaten eggs and cook for 3 minutes.
4. Flip and cook the omelet for 60 seconds more.
5. Fold the omelet into half and cook it more for about half minutes on each side.

Tossed Mango Salsa With Local Bean

Prep time: 30 minutes
Cook time: 1 hour 30 minutes
Servings: 2
Ingredients:
Two fresh limes juice
1 tbsp of organic olive oil
1/4 of one jalapeno – flesh remove and seeded for less "heat" Dice.
1 large tomato half, then spoon out the seeds and watery flesh, then dice the outer flesh. Save for another recipe.
1/8 cup of fresh chopped cilantro
1/2 cup of dried beans, soaked overnight
1/2 peeled and diced mango
Instructions:
1. Bring water to a boil in a skillet, add the soaked beans and simmer until preferred tenderness is achieved, then set aside to cool.
2. Combine together the ingredients in a bowl and toss to coat.
3. Season with fresh cracked black pepper and sea salt to taste.

Oven Roasted Bok Choy

Prep time: 15 minutes
Cook time: 20 minutes
Servings: 6
Ingredients:
Pepper and salt to taste
Extra virgin Olive oil
9 heads of baby bokchoy, cut in half lengthwise
Instructions:
1. Heat up your oven to 450 F.
2. Place the half cut baby bok coy on the baking sheet

3. Drizzle with olive oil lightly, then sprinkle with pepper and salt, toss to coat.
4. Roast coated bok coy for 10 minutes with the cut side down.
5. Flip over and roast for 5 minutes more. Serve with chicken.

Goody Choco Rice Krispies

Prep time: 5 minutes
Cook time: 1 hour
Servings: 8

Ingredients:

1/3 cup of honey
1 tbsp of melted dark chocolate, (optional)
1/2 tsp of pure vanilla extract (optional)
Pinch of salt
1/4 cup of peanut butter
Cups of puffed brown rice cereal, Gluten Free

Instructions:

1. Line an 8"x8" baking sheet using sheets of parchment paper.
2. Combine together all the ingredients in a medium bowl (but reserve the melted chocolate if using) until cereal is well coated.
3. Spread the mixture over the pan evenly and carefully force the mixture down into the pan.
4. Spread a drizzle of melted dark chocolate on top of the bars in the pan.
5. Store in the fridge for at least 60 minutes to set, then remove from the pan, slice, and serve.

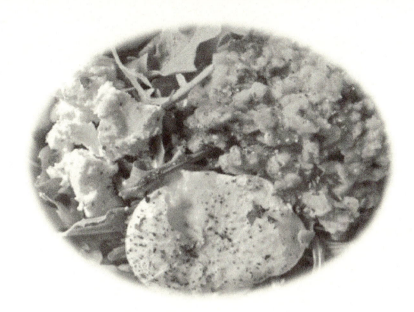

Broccoli Avocado Cucumber Salad

Prep time: 10 minutes
Cook time: 0 minutes
Servings: 4

Ingredients:

1 Cup of cucumber cubes
1 Cup of avocado cubes
2 Cups of blanched broccoli florets
8 tsp of roasted flaxseeds
1 Cup of tomato cubes
2 Cups of iceberg lettuce, torn into pieces
2 Cups of capsicum cubes (yellow, red)

To Be Mixed Into Dressing

4 tbsp olive oil
2 tsp dried mixed herbs
8 tsp lemon juice
Salt and freshly ground black pepper to taste

Instructions:

1. Nicely coat all the ingredients together in a bowl.
2. Mix the dressing ingredients together in another bowl or container.
3. Toss together Just before eating. Eat immediately.

Ocean Breeze Edamame Toss

Prep time: 25 minutes
Cook time: 35 minutes
Servings: 2

Ingredients:
1/8 cup of crumbled reduced-fat feta cheese
1 tablespoons of olive oil
1/2 cup of water
¼ cup of red onion, chopped
1 seeded and chopped medium tomatoes
½ cup of fresh arugula
1/8 teaspoon of fresh ground black pepper
1/2 teaspoon of nicely shredded lemon peel
1 tablespoons of lemon juice
1/2 cup of fresh or frozen, thawed shelled sweet soybeans (ready-to-eat)
1 tablespoons of fresh basil snipped
1/8 teaspoon of salt
1/4 cup of uncooked quinoa, rinsed and drained

Instructions:
1. Boil the quinoa in simmering water in a medium cooking pot, and then reduce the heat. Place the lid on and cook for 15 mins or until liquid is absorbed and quinoa is soft.
2. Add in the edamame when it's about 4-5 minutes before you are through with the cooking.
3. Combine together the chopped tomato, quinoa mixture, onion and arugula in a large bowl.
4. In another small bowl, mix the lemon peel, lemon juice and olive oil together. Add basil, salt, pepper and half of cheese and stir.
3. Add the mixture into the quinoa mixture, toss to coat and spray the remaining half cheese.

Leftover Chicken Anchor Grape Salad

Prep time: 5 minutes
Cook time: 5 minutes
Servings: 2

Ingredients:
1/4 cup of chopped toasted pecans
1 tbsp lemon juice, as dressing
1 tbsp of olive oil
1 large diced ripe tomatoes
1/2 avocado flesh, sliced
1 sliced stalks celery
1/2 cup of red green
1 hard-boiled eggs, sliced
1/2 pounds of cooked leftover chicken

Instructions:
1. Mix together the chicken, toasted pecans, tomatoes, avocado, stalks celery , egg and red green in a large bowl.
2. Drizzle with lemon juice and oil, gently toss to coat well and serve.

Roasted Vegetable Broccoli Pesto Bowls

Prep time: 15 minutes
Cook time: 35 minutes
Servings: 8

Ingredients:

1 teaspoon of garlic powder
4 medium red bell peppers
6 tablespoons of extra-virgin olive oil
6 cups of cooked brown rice
1/2 teaspoon of salt
2 (30 Oz) of can chickpeas
1/2 teaspoon of ground pepper
2 cup of sliced red onion
8 cups of broccoli florets
8 tablespoons of prepared pesto

Instructions:

1. Preheat your oven to 450°F. Mix garlic powder, 3 tablespoons extra-virgin olive oil, salt, pepper and onion together in a large bowl. Add broccoli florets and toss to finely coat.
2. Place in a round baking sheet and roast over medium heat, stir briefly until vegetables are soft, about 20 minutes. Allow the peppers to cool just until you can handle, then chop.
3. Add the remaining 3 tablespoons of oil into rice. Pour in each of eight 2-cup microwave-safe containers about ¾ cup of the cooked brown rice.
4. Divide roasted vegetables and the chickpeas between eight bowls with 1 tablespoon pesto to each.

Chicken Sausage & Red Onion Pasta

Prep time: 30 minutes
Cook time: 30 minutes
Servings: 6

Ingredients:

12 Oz whole-wheat orecchiette pasta or pasta shells
1 1/2 (18 Oz) of sweet Italian chicken sausage links, cut into ¼-inch-thick slices
3/8 teaspoon of pepper
3 tablespoons of extra-virgin olive oil, divided
3/4 teaspoon of salt
3 medium red onions, sliced
10 cups of water

Instructions:

1. Pour cups of water in a large pot to boil over medium-high heat; Heat 1 1/2 tablespoon of oil in a large pan, add the sausage slices and sliced onions, cook stirring frequently until sausage is brown and onion soft (about 10 to 15 minutes).
2. Afterwards, add pasta into the water used to cook the sausage. Cook based on package instructions.
3. Scoop out about 3/4 cup of the cooking water and the drain pasta.
3. Add pasta, sausage and onions into the pan add the 3/8 reserved pasta water and the reserved 1 1/2 tablespoon of oil. Add the remaining cup pasta water in tablespoon measure until desired consistency is reach .Season with the pepper and salt.

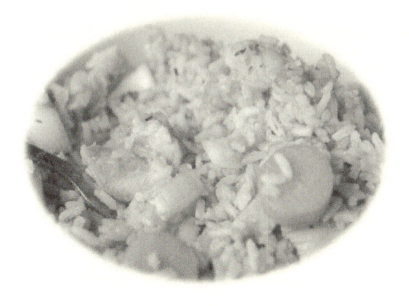

Greek-Way Oregano Chicken Salad

Prep Time: 20 minutes
Cook Time: 20 minutes
Servings: 8

Ingredients:
2 cup of grape tomatoes (halved)
3 cup of chopped cucumber (1 medium)
2 teaspoon of shredded lemon zest
1 teaspoon of dried oregano (crushed)
12 cups of torn romaine lettuce
1 cup of thinly sliced red onion with rings separated
1/2 cup of pitted Kalamata olives, halved
1 cup of vinaigrette salad dressing (Divided into two)
1 cup crumbled reduced-fat feta cheese
4 cups of Shredded Chicken Master Recipe
Lemon wedges for garnish (optional)
1 cup of bottled reduced-calorie Greek
1 1/2 cup of chopped yellow sweet pepper (1 medium)

Instructions:
1. Combine together the lemon zest, chicken, half cup vinaigrette and oregano in a medium bowl and set aside.
2. In a separate large salad bowl, toss the remaining half cup vinaigrette and lettuce. Scoop 1½ cups of romaine lettuce into eight shallow bowls each.
3. Top each bowl with ¼ cup tomatoes, 3 tablespoons of sweet pepper, 2 tablespoons onion and ⅓ cup of chopped cucumber.
4. Drop the chicken mixture into the center of each bowl. Sprinkle with 1 tablespoon olives and 2 tablespoons of feta. Serve with lemon wedges if desired.

DINNER RECIPES

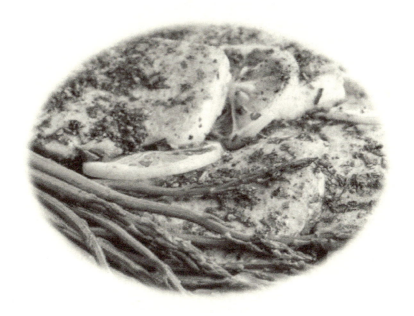

Potato Basil Chickpea Cacciatore

Prep time 25 minutes
Cook time: 45 minutes
Servings: 8

Ingredients:
28 ounces can of crushed tomatoes
2 large sliced red pepper (capsicum)
6 (100g) cups of canned & drained chickpeas or cooked freshly
1 cup of black olives
1 cup (100 g) thickly sliced button mushrooms
2 cup (400 mls) of vegetable stock
2 tablespoon of tomato paste
2 large peeled sweet potato, chopped into bite sizes
2 tablespoon of olive oil
2 handfuls of finely chopped parsley, and more for garnish
8 crushed cloves garlic
2 large handful of finely chopped basil
2 chopped, large brown onions
2 tablespoon of apple cider vinegar

Instructions:
1. Heat 2 tablespoons of olive oil in a broad saucepan over medium-low heat. Add chopped brown onions and garlic and sauté until the onion is tender.
2. Pour in the herbs and sauté for one minute more until fragrant.
3. Add the thinly sliced mushrooms, sweet potato, apple cider vinegar, tomato paste, vegetable stock, and tomatoes. Simmer for 10 minutes, stirring frequently.
4. Stir in the rest of the ingredients; simmer on medium low heat, stirring frequently, for 10 minutes more.
5. Serve with basmati, brown rice or cauliflower rice, and garnish with parsley.

Whole-Wheat Spaghetti Lemon with Salmon

Prep time: 10 minutes
Cook time: 10 minutes
Servings: 2

Ingredients:
1 1/2 tbsp of capers
1 cups of baby spinach leaves, fresh organic
1 tbsp of lemon juice
1/2 lemon, zested
1 tbsp of olive oil (extra-virgin)
2 pieces, Alaskan salmon, wild caught
1/4 tsp of black pepper, freshly ground, plus more
1/4 tsp of salt, plus more
1/8 cup of fresh basil leaves, chopped
1/2 minced garlic clove
1/4 lbs of whole grain pasta
1/2 tbsp of olive oil

Instructions:
1. Cook your pasta according to the package instructions, about 8-10 minutes or until al dente. Drain.
2. Combine together the drained pasta, extra-virgin olive oil, garlic, pepper, and salt in a large bowl. Toss together until well incorporated and set aside.
3. In a medium frying pan, heat the olive oil over medium-high heat.
4. Sprinkle salt and freshly ground pepper on the salmon to season it, then add it to the heated oil in the pan.
5. Cook to your desire, I cooked mine for about 2 minutes on each side based on the fish thickness; Set the salmon aside in a bowl.
6. Combine together the lemon juice, lemon zest, capers, and basil into the spaghetti mix and toss to combine.
7. Arrange 2 serving plates, add a half cup of spinach to each bowl, top with 1/2 pasta, and add a piece of salmon on top of each pasta. Serve immediately.

Mixed Vegetable Meal

Prep time: 20 minutes
Cook time: 15 minutes
Servings: 6

Ingredients:
1 1/2 tsp of cumin seeds
1 1/2 bay leaf
3 whole dry kashmiri red chilies, cut into small sizes
3/4 tsp methi seeds
3/4 tsp of nigella seeds
3/4 tsp of chopped green chilies
1 1/2 cup of French beans, chopped
3/4 tsp of turmeric powder
1 1/2 tsp of mustard seeds
3 tsp of olive oil
1 1/2 cup of green peas
A pinch of sugar and salt to taste
3/4 cup eggplant, cut into 1/2" cubes
1 1/2 cup of red pumpkin cubes
1 1/2 cup of cauliflower florets
3/4 tsp of aniseeds

Instructions:
1. In a deep non-stick skillet, heat 3 teaspoons of olive oil, add the bay leaf, green, nigella seeds, chilies, menti seeds, cumin seeds, aniseeds, mustard seeds and red chilies and sauté for 1 minute over medium heat.
2. Add in 1 cup of water and the remaining ingredients, mix well.
3. Cover and cook for 12 to 14 minutes over a medium heat, stirring not too often. Serve hot.

Baked ChilliLime Chicken

Prep time: 5 minutes
Cook time: 50 minutes
Servings: 6

Ingredients:
3 tbsp of lime juice
Salt and pepper, to taste
1 1/2 tsps of dried chili flakes
3 tsps of grated lime zest
6 tbsp of olive oil
3 pounds of chicken drumsticks
3 crushed cloves garlic

Instructions:
1. Set chicken drumsticks aside in a shallow bowl.
2. Combine together all the ingredients in a bowl and whisk thoroughly until fully combined.
3. Add in the chicken drumsticks, cover and place in the refrigerator for two hours.
4. Heat up the oven to 375 F.
5. Greased an oven tray, and then transfer the chicken drumsticks over the tray.

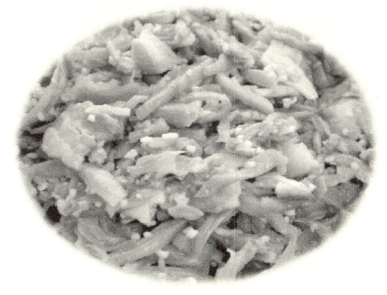

Garlic Cilantro Lime Rice

Prep time: 5 minutes
Cook time: 20 minutes
Servings: 6

Ingredients:

4 cups of long-grain rice
2 tsp of kosher salt
8 cups of low-sodium chicken broth
6 limes Juice and 2 limes zest (reserve 1 lime juice for garnish)
Fresh cilantro, chopped for garnish
2 tbsp of vegetable oil
2 large chopped onions
6 minced cloves garlic

Instructions:

1. Heat 2 tablespoons of vegetable oil over medium heat in a large skillet.
2. Add in the chopped onions and minced garlic and cook until softened, about 3 to 4 minutes.
3. Lower the heat and add the rice; cook, stirring constantly for about 3 minutes, making an effort to ensure that the rice isn't burnt.
4. Add four limes' zest and four lime juice into a liquid measuring cup. Combine the lime juice and chicken broth. This should give you about eight cups.
5. Pour the juice/liquid into the rice, and add salt.
6. Increase your stove temperature to medium heat and bring mixture to a boil, reduce to low heat and simmer with the lid on for 10 to 15 minutes or until the rice is soft. Try and avoid the rice being sticky.
7. To serve, stir more lime juice and chopped cilantro to taste or garnish with lime wedges.

Coconut Zucchinis Curry Fish

Prep time 15 minutes
Cook time: 15 minutes
Servings 4

Ingredients:
4 large chopped zucchinis
2 cups of diced pumpkin
4 crushed cloves garlic
2 tsp of freshly grated ginger
4 cups of fish or vegetable stock
4 tbsp of curry powder
2 (13.25 oz each) can of full fat coconut milk
2 medium diced brown onions.
4 large chopped carrots
2 pounds of white flesh fish, cut into chunks
2 tsp of garam masala
 Salt and pepper to taste

Instructions:
1. Combine all ingredients one after the other, with the exception of the fish, in a large skillet (enough to contain everything) over medium heat. Cook until heated through, then reduce the heat and cook until the carrots are tender to your liking.
2. Add the fish pieces, cook on low heat for about 5 minutes, or until fish easily flakes with a fork. Divide into 4 servings portions and enjoy!

Sweet Potato With Kale Chili Portobello

Prep time 10 minutes
Cook time: 25 minutes
Servings: 4

Ingredients:
375g peeled medium sweet potato, diced into tiny cubes
3/4 tsps of salt
3/8 tsps of paprika or less
3/4 tsp. of cumin
1 1/2 tbsp of coconut oil
1 1/2 cups of vegetable broth
105g cup of chopped kale
 3 chopped portobello mushrooms
21.25oz can of diced tomatoes
4 1/2 chopped garlic cloves

3/8 tsps of chili powder or less
1 1/2 chopped onion
Instructions:
1. Pour 1 1/2 tablespoons of coconut oil into a soup pot, add the chopped garlic and chopped onion, and cook over medium heat for 2 minutes.
2. Add the vegetable broth, paprika, chili powder, sweet potato, mushrooms, diced tomatoes, and salt to taste.
3. Simmer over medium-low heat with the lid on, about 25 minutes until potatoes are soft, stirring not too often. Stir in the kale and cook on medium low heat until kale is wilted.

Sweet Potato With Lentil Bolognese Noodles

Prep time 30 minutes
Cook time: 40 minutes
Servings 6
Ingredients:
375 ml cup of vegetable stock
1 (75 g) cup of fresh basil or 1 1/2 tsp dried
1 1/2 teaspoon of dried rosemary
1 1/2 chopped zucchini
3/8 cup of water
3 medium sweet potatoes, spiralized and blanched
1 1/2 tablespoon of apple cider vinegar
300g of quartered mushrooms
3 tablespoon of tomato paste
1 1/2 tablespoon olive oil
300 g cup of red lentils
4 1/2 crushed garlic cloves
1 1/2 chopped celery stalk
1 1/2 chopped carrot
375 g cup of tomato tomato sauce
1 1/2 large chopped brown onion
1 1/2 teaspoon of dried thyme
Instructions:
1. Heat 1 1/2 tablespoon of olive oil in a saucepan over medium low heat and sauté the onions, celery, carrots and garlic in the hot oil for 5 minutes.
2. Stir in the rest ingredients (but reserve the sweet potato) and simmer until the sauce has thickened and the lentils are cooked through; about 20 minutes.

3. Add the reserved sweet potatoes and steam the potatoes in frying pan, about 3 minutes until soft. Serve with nutritional yeast or vegan parmesan cheese.

Turkey Meatloaf With Tomato Ketchup

Prep time: 15 minutes
Cook time: 1 hour
Servings: 4

Ingredients:
1 large eggs, beaten
Freshly ground black pepper
1/4 tsp of salt
1/8 cup of ketchup
1/2 finely chopped medium onion
4-oz can of zero-salt-added tomato sauce
1/4 cup of orange or red bell pepper, seeded and chopped
1 lbs of lean ground turkey breast
3/8 cup of quick-cooking oats
1/4 cup of nonfat milk
1 tsp of Worcestershire sauce

Instructions:
1. Heat up your oven to 350°F.
2. Start by stirring the milk and oats together in a small bowl. Leave in the bowl to soak up to 3 minutes.
3. Combine together other ingredients in a separate large bowl but reserve the tomato sauce. Stir until fully combined.
4. Pour the mixture into a baking dish and form into a loaf. Spread the reserved tomato sauce on top the meatloaf.
5. Place baking pan in the preheated oven and bake until it reads 160°F when an instant-read thermometer is inserted into the meat center, about 1 hour.
6. Let rest out of the oven for about 10 to 15 minutes before slicing.

Merry Spanakopita

Prep time: 15 minutes
Cook time: 45 minutes
Serves: 6

Ingredients:
1 1/2 tablespoon of chopped fresh dill
Handful of chopped fresh parsley leaves
3 tablespoon of coconut milk or Greek yogurt
1 1/2 teaspoon of sea salt
3 tablespoon of lemon juice
3/4 teaspoon of cracked black pepper
3/4 cup of pitted olives chopped in half
3 tablespoon of parmesan cheese (optional)
1 1/2 (150g) small bunch of kale — strip off the stems and leaves and chop finely
1 1/2 tablespoon of olive or coconut oil
3/4 (450g) bunch of finely chopped Swiss chard, including some stems
3 crushed garlic cloves
1 1/2 sliced leek
6 eggs

Instructions:
1. Heat up your oven to 350°F.
2. Heat 1 1/2 tablespoon of your preferred oil in a saucepan over medium heat. Add crushed garlic and sliced leek and cook for about 60 seconds until tender. Add in the fresh chopped dill, kale and Swiss chard. Cook on low heat, stirring often until spinach has wilted, about 5 minutes. Drain.
3. Combine together the remaining ingredients, stir in the kale mixture and stir well to incorporate everything. Transfer into a greased pie dish and place in the oven and bake for 45 minutes.
4. Sprinkle with the parmesan cheese before baking (Optional).
5. Serve beside salad and lemon wedges.

Zucchinis Mushrooms, Fettuccini Alfredo

Prep time: 30 minutes
Cook time: 90 minutes
Servings: 2

Ingredients:
For the Alfredo sauce:
½ teaspoon of lemon juice
¼ teaspoon of cracked pepper
½ tablespoon of nutritional yeast
¼ teaspoon of sea salt
½ sliced leek
3 tablespoon of water
2 finely chopped garlic cloves
½ small cauliflower head, chopped into florets
1/8 cup of cashew, soaked in hot water for an hour, rinse
½ tablespoon of coconut oil
For the dish:
½ handful of parsley
1 large zucchinis
½ tablespoon of coconut oil
½ (150g) cup of thickly sliced button mushrooms

Instructions:
1. Add 3 tablespoon of water along with the cauliflower in a medium saucepan, Cook for 10 minutes with the lid on until tender, Drain.
2. Heat ½ tablespoon of coconut oil in a medium frying pan over medium-low heat; Sauté the leek and garlic until soft for 5 minutes.
3. Blend the drained cauliflower, soaked cashews, yeast, salt, lemon juice, pepper, sautéed leeks and water in a blender that can hold everything until smooth.
4. Use a vegetable spiralizer to spiralize the zucchini into thick ribbons.
5. Fry the sliced mushrooms in the same fry pan used to sauté the leek and garlic with the coconut oil still inside, until golden brown. Stir in the cauliflower Alfredo sauce and zucchini fettuccine and cook until heated through. Served garnish with parsley.

DESSERTS RECIPES

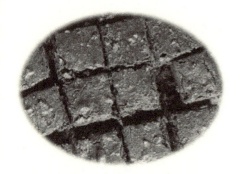

Vanilla Cashew Bites

Prep time: 5 minutes
Cook time: 5 minutes
Servings: 6 muffins

Ingredients:
1 tablespoon of coconut oil
1/2 tsp of vanilla extract
1/2 tablespoon of inulin powder
1/2 cup of cashews
Pinch of salt
1/8 cup of unflavored protein powder
10 drops of stevia liquid

Instructions:
1. Blend all the ingredients together in a food processor until well combined and smooth.
2. Pour mixture into 6 mini muffin cups lined with mini cupcake papers. Place in the freezer to set. Serve cold and store in an airtight container.

Oats With Peanut ButterGranola Bars

Prep time: 5 minutes
Cook time: 1 hour
Servings: 9

Ingredients:
3/8 cup of cacao nibs
2 cups of quick cooking rolled oats
1 1/2 cups of peanut butter (homemade)
3/8 cup of sliced almonds
3/8 teaspoon of vanilla essence
3 tablespoons of roasted flax seeds
1 1/2 tablespoon of coconut oil
Pinch of salt
3 tablespoons of honey or maple syrup

Instructions:
1. Arrange a deep mixing bowl, and mix all the ingredients together in the bowl until finely combined and smooth.
2. Line a grease-proofpaper on a tray, pour in the mixture, and press out using a silicon scapula or palm to form a square.
3. Place in the refrigerator for no less than an hour. Remove and cut into rectangles of 9 equal bars.
4. Store in the refrigerator in an air-tight container for up to 1 week.

Quick Starter Lime Mousse

Prep time: 5 minutes
Cook time: 1 minute
Servings: 8

Ingredients:
2 tbsp of maple syrup
2 tsp of lime zest
2 tbsp of coconut oil
2 bananas
4 large avocados
1/2 cup of lime juice, fresh squeezed

Instructions:
1. Chill the avocados without pilling for one hour in the refrigerator.
2. Peel avocado, pit and add it to the blender along with the coconut oil, maple syrup, lime juice, and banana; blend for up to 60 seconds. Serve garnish with lime zest.

Yankee Spicy Stewed Apples

Prep time: 15 minutes
Cook time: 30 minutes
Servings: 8

Ingredients:
2 teaspoon of ground cinnamon or more
2 teaspoons of maple syrup or honey (if desired)
1/2 cup of water
8 apples, remove core and chopped
1 teaspoon of ground nutmeg
1/2 teaspoon of ground ginger or more

Instructions:
1. Combine all the ingredients in a medium pot and heat until it simmers.
2. Reduce to low heat, stir everything together, and cook for about 30 minutes, or until the apples are tender.
3. Stir frequently and add water in case the mixture becomes too dry.
4. To serve, dollop canned coconut cream.

Quick Cheese Prosciutto Peaches

Prep time: 10 minutes
Cook time: 10 minutes
Servings: 4

Ingredients:
2 large ripe peaches, (halved and pitted)
4 tsps of honey
Chopped fresh mint (for garnish)
4 thinly slices prosciutto
2 oz soft goat cheese

Instructions:
1. Warm-up your grill for a medium heat. Add ½ oz of the goat cheese inside each peach half.
2. Wrap a slice of prosciutto around each peach half and press a little.
3. Oil grill rack and grill each wrapped peaches, covered, turning occasionally until the prosciutto is crisp and brown. Mine took about 6 minutes. If desired, sprinkle with mint and drizzle with

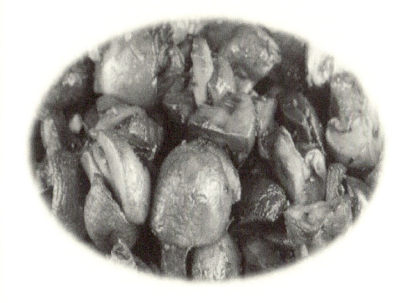

Plum Nut Almond CrumbleMuffin

Prep time: 10 minutes
Cook time: 20 minutes
Servings: 4

Ingredients:
30 g cup of buckwheat or chopped pecans, or almonds
42.5 g cup of chopped walnuts
1 tablespoons of maple syrup
Plums, slice in half and remove seed
30.2 g cup of almond meal
2 tablespoons of coconut oil, slightly hardened

Instructions:
1. Heat up your oven to 350F.
2. Start by scooping out some of the plum flesh into a bowl.
3. Add rest ingredients in the bowl and use your fingers to rub in the coconut oil until mixture is well combined.
3. Add the mixture over the plums and place in a baking tray lined with parchment paper.
4. Bake in the preheated oven until the plums are tender, about 15 to 20 minutes.

Mango Vanilla Tiramisù

Prep time: 30 minutes
Cook time: 8 h 30 minutes
Servings: 4

Ingredients:
1/2 cup of frozen light whipped topping, thawed
1/2 cup of nonfat vanilla Greek yogurt
1/8 teaspoon of almond extract
1 cubed medium mangoes, or 8 ounces of both frozen or refrigerated mango and more for garnish
1 tablespoons of light agave syrup
6 crisp lady fingers, break into 1-inch pieces

Instructions:
1. Divide the mango cubes into two and place half of the cubes into a food processor, process until smooth.
2. Transfer the mango puree into a small bowl. Stir in the almond extract and agave syrup. Add the mango cubes that were reserved into the food processor and process until its coarsely chopped, then set aside.
3. Carefully wrap your thawed whipped topping into nonfat vanilla Greek yogurt in another small bowl.
3. Divide the ladyfinger pieces into two and spread one portion into a baking dish and spoon half of the yogurt mixture and half of the mango puree over them.
4. Top it with the chopped mango. Add the remaining half of the ladyfinger pieces on top. Layer the puree and yogurt on the remaining ladyfingers, Cover tiramisu with plastic wrap.
4. Refrigerate for about 8 to 24 hours until the ladyfingers are softened. Serve cold, if desired garnished with mango.

Orange Cherry Crisp

Prep time: 25 minutes
Cook time: 25 minutes
Servings: 3

Ingredients:
1 tablespoons of ground flaxseed
1/2 Orange
1 tablespoons of unsalted butter, melted
1/2 teaspoon of ground cinnamon
1 tablespoon of sliced almonds
1/4 cup of old-fashioned rolled oats
1/8 cup of almond flour
1/2 tablespoon of cornstarch
1/8 cup of sweetener
1/2 pound of frozen or fresh unsweetened pitted cherries

Instructions:
1. Grate about 1/2 tablespoon zest from orange and juice the orange to get about ¼ cup of liquid. Set the juice and zest aside.
2. Heat a heavy skillet or an 8-inch cast-iron over a medium heat. Add in the oats and cook to toast, stirring occasionally like 3 minutes.
3. Add the melted butter, almond flour, almonds, brown sugar, cinnamon and flaxseed.
4. Cook and stir regularly for 60 seconds until coarse crumbs is formed. (Be mindful, the topping can get brown very quick.) Transfer into a bowl.
5. Combine the cornstarch and cherries together in the skillet. Stir in the juice and reserved orange zest and cook over a medium-high heat, stir frequently until thick and also bubbly.
6. Cook and stir for about 2 additional minutes. Sprinkle your reserved topping on the cherry mixture.

Pineapple Mango Lemon Cream

Prep time; 5 minutes
Cook time: 5 minutes
Servings: 12

Ingredients:
2 cup of frozen or fresh mango chunks
2 tablespoon of lemon or lime juice
32-oz package of frozen pineapple chunks

Instructions:
1. Process lemon or lime juice, pineapple and mango in a food processor until it's smooth and creamy. Add 1 cup of water if using frozen mango. Best serve immediately.

Pecan Peanut Butter Banana Cake

Prep time: 10 minutes
Cook time: 1 hour
Serves: 6

Ingredients:
3/4 cup of almond meal
1 1/2 tsp of baking soda
1 1/2 tsp of cinnamon
3/8 cup of pecans, chopped
6 ripe, mashed bananas
6 tbsp of coconut oil, softened
1 1/2 tsp of baking powder
3/4 cup of peanut butter
6 eggs, whisked
1 1/2 tsps of ground cloves

Instructions:
1. Heat up your oven to 350 F. Whisk together the peanut butter, eggs and mashed bananas in a blender and blend until you have a fine smooth mixture.
2. In a medium mixing bowl, mix together all the ingredients with hand until combined.
3. Greased a cake tin with coconut oil and Pour in the mixture.
4. Place into the cake tin in preheated oven and bake for one hour or until toothpick inserted in the center of the cake comes out clean.
5. Refrigerate the cake in an airtight container.

SALADS RECIPES

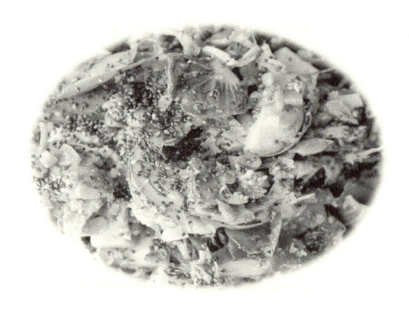

Beets Steamed Edamame Salad

Prep time: 15 minutes
Cook time: 5 minutes
Servings: 8

Ingredients:
2 bag of steamed edamame beans
White vinegar
20-24 oz. can of beets
4 teaspoon of olive oil of high quality
12 large organic carrots, cubed
6 corn on the cobs, corn cut off
Black pepper
1 pound of green beans cut in 1 inch segments

Instructions:
1. Wet a paper towel and wrapped the corn with the damp towel; place the wrapped corn in the microwave for 5 minutes.
2. Steam the entire ingredients (reserving corn and beets) in large steamer in this other; carrots cubes, green beans, and edamame beans on the top layer.
3. Mix beets together with the cooked corn and cooked vegetables.
4. Toss salad slightly with a few dashes of black pepper, white vinegar and olive oil.

Avocado Cilantro Chunky Salsa

Prep time: 10 minutes
Cook time: 0 minutes
Servings: 6

Ingredients:
6 tbsp of chopped cilantro leaves
3 tbsp of avocado or macadamia nut oil
3 large diced ripe tomato
1 ½ finely diced spring onion
3 large diced avocado
Salt and pepper
6 tbsp of lime juice

Instructions:
1. Add the entire ingredients together in a bowl and carefully toss. Serve it right away.

Potatoes Mixed Vegetables

Prep time: 10 minutes
Cook time: 1 hour 20 minutes
Servings: 12

Ingredients:
12 thinly sliced medium tomatoes
2 tbsp of dried oregano
2 cup water
2 1/2 cups of tomato passata or tomato puree
1 cup of extra-virgin olive oil, plus more if needed
4 tbsp of finely chopped flat-leaf parsley
10 sliced into rounds small zucchini
2 thinly sliced large onion
24 cherry tomatoes
6 sliced garlic cloves
2 large eggplant, sliced lengthwise and cut into half round thick slices
Salt and fresh ground pepper
3 lbs (about 8 medium) potatoes cut into 1/2 inch cube

Instructions:
1. Heat up your oven to 425 F.
2. Pour about four tablespoons of olive oil in a saucepan over medium heat, cook the eggplant in hot oil in batches for about 5–7 minutes, (you can add more oil if needed) until the eggplants are golden and softened; Set aside in a bowl.
3. Add the sliced garlic cloves and sliced onion into the pan used for cooking eggplants. Sauté until fragrant and softened, about 5 minutes. Set aside in the same bowl as the eggplants.
4. Add two cups of water, potato cubes, passata, zucchini and tomatoes to the bowl. Sprinkle on top with the chopped parsley leaf and oregano; Season with ground black pepper and salt. Mix very well to fully combine, then transfer to a broad ovenproof dish. Drizzle with oil.
5. Place in the preheated oven and bake for 30 minutes.
6. Reduce oven heat to 400 F and bake for 20–30 minutes extra, or until the vegetables are tender and top is brown. Let cool a bit before serving.

Toasted Mango Pepitas Kale Salad

Prep time: 20 minutes
Cook time: 0 minutes
Servings 8

Ingredients:
4 tsps of honey
2 fresh mango, thinly diced (about 1 cup)
Freshly ground black pepper
4 full tbsp of toasted pepitas
Kosher salt
One lemon juice
2 large bunch of kale de-stalk and sliced into ribbons
1/2 cup of extra-virgin olive oil, plus more

Instructions:
1. Add the sliced kale into a large mixing bowl; add half the lemon juice and little salt.
2. Start working on the kale using your fingertips for five minutes, or until the kale leaves are tender and sweet.
3. Spread olive oil over the kale and work on the kale with your finger for few more minute. Set aside.
4. Blend the black pepper, honey with the remaining half lemon juice in a small bowl.
5. Steadily drip in 1/2 cup of olive oil while whisking until it forms a dressing. Season dressing with a pinch of salt.
5. Pour few dressing on the kale, and add the pepitas and mango. Toss together and serve.

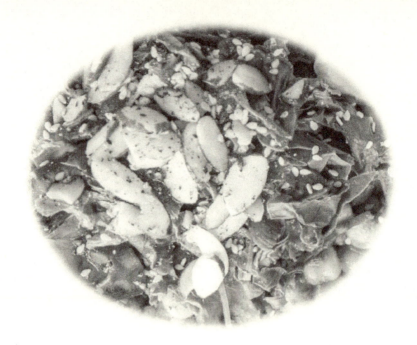

Chickpea And Parsley Pumpkin Salad

Prep time: 5 minutes
Cook time: 10 minutes
Servings: 6

Ingredients:
1 1/2 small thinly sliced red onion
1 1/2 handfuls parsley, chopped
1 1/2 diced avocado
1 1/2 tbsp of lemon juice
1 1/2 tsp of ground coriander
1 1/2 tsp of ground cumin
Salt and pepper, to season
3 tbsp of olive oil
1 1/2 cups of pumpkin, peeled and chopped into bite pieces
1 1/2 (21.5 oz) can of chickpeas, rinsed and drained

Instructions:
1. Season the pumpkin with a drizzle of olive oil, coriander and cumin on top.
2. Arrange seasoned pumpkin in an oven tray lined with parchment paper.
3. Roast until the pumpkin is lightly browned and soft.
4. Combine the salad ingredients into a bowl, and then drizzle in lemon juice.

White Bean Cherry Tomatoes Cucumber Salad

Prep time: 10 minutes
Cook Time: 10 minutes
Servings: 3

Ingredients:
1 ½ avocado, diced
Cherry tomatoes and chopped cucumbers
1 Cup of canned white beans, rinsed and drained
6 teaspoons of extra-virgin olive oil
3 tablespoons of red-wine vinegar
3/4 cup of crumbled feta cheese
3/4 cup of chopped red onion
Freshly ground pepper to taste
6 cups of mixed salad greens
3/4 teaspoon of kosher salt

Instructions:
1. Combine beans, veggies, avocado and greens in a medium bowl.
2. Season with salt and pepper.
3. Drizzle with vinegar and oil, combine by tossing, then transfer into a large plate.

Arugula Cucumber Tuna Salad

Prep time: 5 minutes
Cook time: 5 minutes
Servings: 4

Ingredients:
1 tsp of dried oregano
2 tbsp of lemon juice
4 tbsp of olive oil
12 oz can of tuna, drained
2 handfuls of arugula leaves
1 sliced Lebanese cucumber
2 small coarsely grated zucchini
1 cup of cherry tomatoes, halved

Instructions:
1. In a medium mixing bowl, combine all the salad ingredients. Drizzle with lemon juice and olive oil. Enjoy!

Springtime Chicken Berries Salad

Prep time: 5 minutes
Cook time: 5 minutes
Servings: 8

Ingredients:

Salad:

4 cups of quartered strawberries
2/3 cup of vertically sliced red onion
2 cup of fresh blueberries
24 oz of boneless, skinless, rotisserie chicken breast, sliced
8 cups of arugula
8 cups of torn romaine lettuce

Dressing:

2 tbsp of water
2/8 tsps of freshly ground black pepper
2/8 tsps of salt
4 tbsp of extra-virgin olive oil
4 tbsp of red wine vinegar
2 tbsp of low carb sweetener of your choice

Instructions:

1. In a large mixing bowl, combine together the blueberries, strawberries, arugula, romaine and onions. Toss gently to combine. "
2. Combine together 2 tbsp of water, black pepper, red wine vinegar, salt, and sweetener in a small bowl. Fold in the olive oil, stirring often until well incorporated.
3. Arrange eight different plates and place up to 2 cups of chicken mixture on each. Drizzle with 4 teaspoons of the dressing.

Toaster Almond Spiralized Beet Salad

Prep time: 15 minutes
Cook time: 15 minutes
Servings: 4

Ingredients:
1/8 teaspoon of ground pepper
1/8 cup of extra-virgin olive oil
1/4 teaspoon of freshly grated lemon zest
1 pounds beets (2 medium)
1/4 cup of (fresh) chopped flat-leaf parsley
1 tablespoons of lemon juice
1/4 cup of slivered almonds, toasted
1/4 teaspoon of salt
1/6 cup of minced shallot

Instructions:
1. Mix together the minced shallot, lemon juice, oil, salt, pepper and lemon zest into a small bowl. Mix gently to combine then set aside.
2. Peel the beets with a thin blade, then spiralize and cut into 3-inch lengths.
3. Arrange the spiralized beets into a large bowl. Sprinkle beets on top with the dressing, toss gently to make sure the salad is finely coated.
4. Add chopped parsley and almonds before serving. Toss to coat.

SOUPS RECIPES

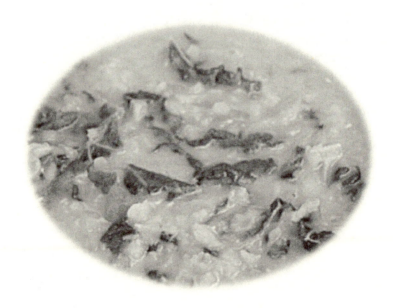

Apple Leeks Mascarpone Soup

Prep time: 5 minutes
Cook time: 35 minutes
Servings: 3

Ingredients:
1/2 cup of chopped leeks
Salt and pepper
Nutmeg to taste
1 cored, peeled and diced apple
1.5 lbs of butternut squash, peeled and cubed
1/2 chopped medium onion
1 tbsp of unsalted butter
3 cups of chicken stock

For the Mascarpone Topping:
1 tablespoons of milk
1/4 teaspoon of cinnamon
1/4 cup of mascarpone cheese

Instructions:
1. Melt butter over medium heat in a large pot. Add apples, leeks, and onions. Cook about 8 minutes until soft and translucent.
2. Add chicken stock into the pot along with squash and cook until heated through, then simmer on low heat for about 20 to 25 minutes until squash is tender. Set aside.
3. Mascarpone topping: In the meantime, combine together the 3 last ingredients and stir until totally combined. Set aside.
4. Blend soup using an immersion blender or puree in a blender and transfer back to the pot.
5. Stir well and season the soup with pepper nutmeg and salt.
6. Pour soup into bowls and serve with a dollop of mascarpone topping in the middle.

Aminos Mushroom Soup

Prep time: 10 minutes
Cook time: 35 minutes
Servings: 8

Ingredients:
4 dried bay leaves
Black pepper, freshly ground
4 tablespoons of tapioca flour
4 cups of unsweetened almond or cashew milk
4 cups of organic vegetable broth
2 tsp salt
40 stalks of fresh thyme, leaves removed
20 oz packages of sliced baby portobello mushroom
4 large diced white onions
20 oz packages of sliced white button mushroom
2 tablespoon of liquid aminos

Instructions:
1. Sweat the diced onions dry for about 5 to 7 minutes in a large non-stick saucepan over medium heat.
2. Shift the onions towards the sides of the saucepan, add mushrooms slices to the middle of the saucepan, and cook for 5 minutes without covering.
3. Mix both ingredients together, add in the thyme and keep cooking, about 10 minutes or more.
4. Add the liquid aminos, bay leaf and salt to the mushrooms onion mixture.
5. Mix the vegetable broth and tapioca starch in a small mixing bowl until no more lumps and well combined. Pour the mixture into the mushrooms and stir, then add almond milk.
6. Cook about 15 minutes, stirring once in a while until heated through. Adjust taste with freshly ground black pepper. You can add Parmesan cheese, cashew cheese if desired.

Detox-Liver Arugula And Broccoli Soup

Prep time: 3 minutes
Cook time: 20 minutes
Servings: 4

Ingredients:
5 cups of water
2 cup of arugula leaves, packed
1/2 teaspoon of dried thyme
1/2 teaspoon of freshly ground black pepper
2 tablespoon olive oil
1/2 teaspoon of salt
1 lemon Juice
1 yellow or Spanish onion, roughly diced
2 clove of garlic, chopped
2 (about 4/6 pounds) head broccoli, cut into little florets

Instructions:
1. Heat 2 tablespoon of olive oil over medium in a large saucepan. Cook onion in the heated oil until soft and translucent.
2. Pour in chopped garlic and cook for 60 seconds, add broccoli and keep cooking for about 4 minutes more or until it is bright green. Add 1/2 teaspoon of freshly ground black pepper, salt, thyme and cups of water. Allow mixture to heat through, lower heat and cook with the lid on for about 8 minutes or until broccoli is tender.
3. Blend the soup in a blender or use an immersion blender. Add the arugula, blend until smooth. Serve with lemon juice.

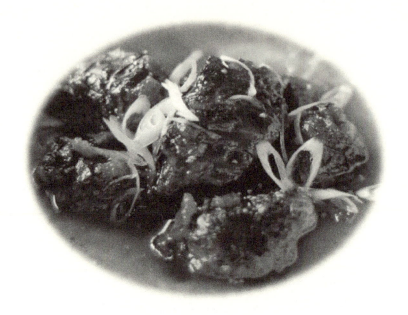

Unique Lentil with KaleSoup

Prep time: 10 minutes
Cook time 1 hour 10 minutes
Servings: 2

Ingredients
1/2 cup of wild rice
1/2 cup of steel cut oats or barley
1/2 cup of lentils (any will do)
4 cups of kale, chopped
1/2 cup of French lentils
8 cups of vegetarian broth

Instructions:
1. Cook the vegetarian broth in a soup pot over medium heat until heated through and add the other ingredients, stir.
2. Simmer on low with the lid on for 45 minutes to 1 hour.
3. Add chopped kale, stir, and simmer for 10 more minutes. Serve and enjoy.

Pasta Veggies Minestrone Soup

Prep time: 15 minutes
Cook time: 40 minutes
Servings: 2-4

Ingredients:
1 tbsp basil, finely chopped or 1 tsp of dried basil
1 minced garlic cloves
14 ounce can of diced plum tomatoes
1/8 tsp of salt
1/8 cup of your preferred pasta
1/16 tsp black pepper, freshly ground
3/8 cup of diced celery
1/2 cup of cannellini beans
1.5 cups of water
1/2 cup of carrots, peeled and sliced
1 cups of diced zucchini
3/8 cup of chopped onion
1/2 tbsp of extra virgin olive oil
1/8 tsp of dried oregano

Instructions:
1. Heat-up a saucepan over medium heat.
2. Drizzle a saucepan with olive oil and sauté the chopped onion, about 4 minutes, stirring periodically until browned a bit. Without the pasta, add in the rest ingredients and bring to a boil.
3. Reduce to low heat and simmer with the lid on for 25 minutes, stirring occasionally.
4. Add and cook pasta according to package instructions, about 10-12 minutes until pasta is al dente.

Pear Red Pepper Soup

Prep time: 10 minutes
Cook time: 40 minutes
Servings: 4-5

Ingredients:
1 sliced shallots
1/4 tsp of dried crushed red pepper
1 (16-oz.) container of no-fat chicken broth
1/4 tsp of ground black pepper
Pinch of ground red pepper
1 peeled and sliced Anjou pears
1 tbsp of butter

1 1/2 large sliced red bell peppers
1 tsp of olive oil
1/8 tsp of salt
Garnishes (optional): fresh thinly sliced pears, chopped fresh chives, plain yogurt.
1 sliced carrots

Instructions:
1. Melt the olive oil with 1 tablespoon of butter over medium heat in a Dutch oven; add the bell pepper, carrots, shallots, and Anjou pears and sauté until tender, about 8 to 10 minutes.
2. Stir in chicken broth and all the peppers, add salt. Cook until heated through. Cover with a lid and simmer on low heat for 25 to 30 minutes. Allow cooling for 20 minutes.
3. In the bowl of a food processor, add and process the soup in batches until smooth, scraping the sides down as necessary. Transfer back to Dutch oven to keep warm until you are ready to use. Garnish, if desired.

Low Heat Chicken Provençal

Prep time: 5 minutes
Cook time: 8 hours
Servings: 8

Ingredients:
1/4 tsp of freshly ground black pepper
2 (16 oz each) can of cannellini beans, rinsed and drained
2 tsp of dried thyme
2 diced red pepper
2 diced yellow pepper
2 (14.5-oz each) can of petite diced tomatoes with basil, oregano and garlic, undrained
1/4 tsp of salt
4 tsp of dried basil
12 oz (skins removed) bone-in chicken breast halves

Instructions:
1. Arrange the chicken into a crock pot; add the rest ingredients into the pot.
2. Cook with the lid on for 8 hours on low-heat setting.

Danny's Tortellini Soup

Prep time: 8 minutes
Cook time: 25 minutes
Servings: 3

Ingredients
1/2 peeled and diced potato
6-6 oz fresh tortellini or frozen (meat or cheese filled)
1 quarts of low sodium chicken stock
2 scallions
1/2 large can of crushed tomatoes (Spice the tomatoes with oregano and basil)
1 tbsp of olive oil
1 medium carrots, peeled and diced
1 small diced zucchini
Black pepper, to taste
1/4 teaspoon of salt
1 diced celery stalks

Instructions:
1. Heat 1 tablespoon of olive oil over medium in a large saucepan. Add in the scallions, diced potatoes, diced celery, carrots, and diced zucchini.
2. Sauté the vegetables for 10 minutes over medium heat, stirring frequently until the vegetables are starting to soften. Add the tomatoes, chicken stock and salt. Flame heat up and bring to a low boil.
3. Add the tortellini and cook about two minutes, then simmer on low heat for 5 to 6 minutes more. Stir in the pepper.

Wellness Parsnip Soup

Prep time: 10 minutes
Cook time: 20 minutes
Serves: 6

Ingredients:
3/4 cup of chopped pumpkin
Salt and pepper, to taste
1 1/2 tsps of ground cumin
7 1/2 cups of stock or broth
6 chopped medium parsnips
1 1/2 tbsp of dried oregano
1 1/2 tbsp of olive oil
4 1/2 crushed garlic cloves
1 1/2 finely chopped brown onion
3 chopped medium carrots

Instructions:
1. Heat 1 1/2 tablespoons of olive oil over medium heat in a large skillet. Sauté the onion and garlic in the pan for about 5 minutes until softened. Mix in the remaining ingredients, reserving only the broth or stock.
2. Cook and stir every now and then for 2 minutes. Add stock or broth and cook until the soup is heated through. Simmer over low heat until the vegetables are tender. Puree the soup with an immersion blender, serve and enjoy.

Feel Good Chicken Soup

Prep time: 10 minutes
Cook time: 10-15 minutes
Serves: 6

Ingredients:
3 large diced carrots
3 bay leaves
1 1/2 medium diced swede or turnip
3 sliced stalks celery
3 tsps of dried oregano
1 1/2 large sliced zucchini
3 tbsp of olive oil
7 1/2 cups of bone stock or broth
6 cups of leftover cooked chicken, shredded
1 1/2 cup of canned coconut cream
Salt and pepper
1 1/2 small diced brown onion

Instructions:
1. Add 3 tablespoons of olive oil in a large pot, sauté the vegetables until they are soft to your liking.
2. Add the remaining ingredients to the pot, reserving the coconut cream. When the vegetables are tender as desired, add in coconut cream and stir to combine.
Turn heat off, garnish with parsley.

SNACKS RECIPES

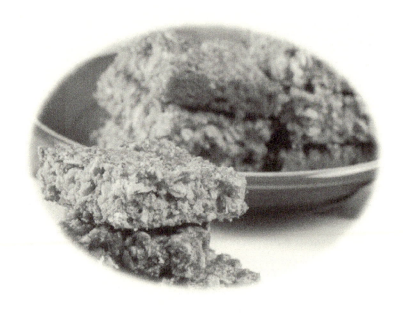

Boneless Chicken Guacamole

Prep time: 30 minutes
Cook time: 50 minutes
Servings: 8

Ingredients:
16-oz boneless, skinless chicken breasts, halved
1 teaspoon of garlic powder
4 tablespoons of chopped fresh cilantro
1 teaspoon of Ground pepper
4 teaspoons of chopped pimientos
1 cup of shredded Monterey Jack cheese (2 ounce)
1 teaspoon of Salt
2 tablespoon of extra-virgin olive oil
2 teaspoon of lime juice
2 medium avocados

Instructions:
1. Gently mash avocado with a fork in a medium bowl until smooth and small chunks remaining.
2. Stir in 2 teaspoon of lime juice, chopped pimientos, a pinch of salt and pepper then Set aside.
3. Sprinkle the chicken with 1 teaspoon of salt, 1 teaspoon pepper and garlic powder.
2. Heat 2 tablespoon of extra-virgin oil in a frying pan over a medium-high heat, add chicken then reduce heat to medium. Turn briefly to cook through, 5 to 6 minutes per side.
3. Top the chicken with cheese, cover to cook more until the cheese melts, about 3 minutes.
4. Place the chicken in serving plates, top with the guacamole and Garnish it with cilantro.

Easy Fresh Guacamole

Prep time: 15 minutes
Cook time: 15 minutes
Servings: 2-3

Ingredients:
6 tbsp of chopped fresh cilantro
6 minced garlic cloves
4 plum tomatoes, seeded and diced
6 ripe Haas avocados
2 pinch of ground cayenne pepper (if desired)
2 small diced red onions
2 teaspoon of salt
2 lime

Instructions:
1. Slice the avocados in half, remove the pits, then spoon avocado out into a bowl. Set one pit aside.
2. Slice through the avocados with a knife (just until your desired consistency is reached) in the bowl.
3. Squeeze the lime to bring out the juice and add into the bowl containing the avocados. Add garlic, tomatoes, cilantro, onion, salt and cayenne pepper (if desired) and stir carefully to combine. While mixing, avoid turning the avocado into a paste.
4. To avoid the avocados becoming brown, place the reserved pit into the avocado or serve immediately with pita chips or tortillas.
5. Cover the bowl with plastic wrap and prevent air from getting inside, refrigerate up to 24 hours.

Garlic Chili Pita Chips

Prep time: 5 minutes
Cook time: 8 minutes
Servings: 3

Ingredients:
Pinch of Garlic powder
3 whole wheat pitas (with pocket or without)
Pinch of Chili powder
Pinch of Salt
1 tsps of olive oil

Instructions:
1. Heat up your oven to 400ºF.
2. Slice each of the individual whole wheat pita in half, then into 4 wedges. Place the pitas onto a broad baking sheet, making sure they do not overlap.
3. Lightly mist the pitas using the olive oil with an oil mister; this will allow the spices to stick or lightly brush the pitas with oil.
4. Sprinkle the pita wedges with the garlic powder, chili powder and salt.
5. Place baking sheet in the preheated oven and bake about 8 minutes or until lightly golden. Serve with, dip, Pico de Gallo or hummus.

Hearty Masala Lotus Seed

Prep time: 2 minutes
Cook time 8 minutes
Servings: 6 cups

Ingredients:
1 teaspoon of cumin seeds powder
2 teaspoon of chaat masala
2 tablespoon of oil
1 teaspoon of chilli powder
6 cups of lotus seeds
Salt

Instructions:
1. Start by dry roasting your lotus seeds in a non-stick frying pan, over medium heat for about 5 minutes. Pour the roasted lotus seeds in a bowl, set aside.
2. In the same pan used in roasting, add two tablespoon of oil, add chaat masala, cumin seeds powder, red chilli powder, and salt to taste, stir well.
3. Heat the pan over medium heat; add roasted lotus seed to other ingredients, stir and sauté for 2 to 3 minutes.
5. You can store in an airtight or Serve immediately.

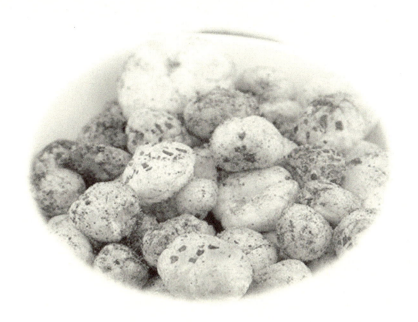

Roasted Spiced Chickpeas Crispy

Prep time: 5 minutes
Cook time: 50 minutes
Servings: 3

Ingredients:
1 tbsp of extra-virgin olive oil
7.5-oz cans of chickpeas, drained and rinsed
1/4 tsp of salt
1/4 teaspoon of dried spices (optional)

Instructions:
1. Heat up the oven to 400°F
2. Spread the drained chickpeas on a baking sheet, leave it without covering. Place in the refrigerator overnight so they will dry out or dry them thoroughly on paper towels.
3. Add 1/4 teaspoon of dried spices to the olive oil to add flavor. Toast the chickpeas with 1 tbsp of olive oil on a baking sheet until well coated. Sprinkle with salt. Toss once more then spread out on the baking sheet evenly.
4. Place in the preheated oven and bake for about 50 minutes to 1 hour or until crispy, shake the pan every 5-10 minutes so the chickpeas will be crisp evenly.
5. Allow to cool down at room temperature. Serve and enjoy!

HoneyNut Raisins Granola

Prep time: 3 minutes
Cook time: 25 minutes
Servings:

Ingredients:
3/8 cup of honey
1/2 tsp of pure vanilla extract
1 tsp of ground cinnamon
1/8 tsp of salt
2 cups of old-fashioned rolled oats
1/2 cup golden or red raisins
1 cups nuts, coarsely chopped
1/4 cup of butter

Instructions:
1. Preheat the oven to 350 F.
2. Combine together the raisins, chopped nuts and oats in a large bowl.
3. Combine together the vanilla, ground cinnamon, butter, honey and salt in a saucepan over medium heat; bring to a boil for about 60 seconds.
4. Gently toss the oat/nut mixture and the honey mixture together until finely coated.
5. Spread the mixture evenly onto a greased cookie sheet.
6. Place the cookie sheet in the preheated oven and bake until lightly browned, about 20 minutes; stirring every 5 minutes and then spreading back to even layer. Allow granola cooling out of the oven, then crumble. Can be stored up to 2 weeks in an airtight container.

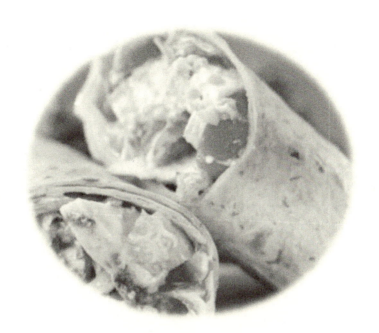

Cornmeal Cauliflower Fritters

Prep time: 5 minutes
Cook time 25-35 minutes
Servings: 5 Fritters

Ingredients:
1/4 teaspoon of fresh ground black pepper
2 1/2 tablespoon of nutritional yeast
1/6 cup of flour
1/2 medium size head of cauliflower, break
2 tablespoon of cornmeal
1 large egg
3/8 teaspoon of salt
Coconut oil
1 minced garlic cloves
1/4 teaspoon of chili powder
1 tablespoon of fresh chopped cilantro

Instructions:
1. Cook cauliflower florets for 5 minutes in a saucepan over medium heat. Drain and chop into tiny pieces while still warm.
2. Stir the cooked cauliflower with salt, pepper, cilantro, garlic and chili powder.
3. Crack the egg and whisk in a separate bowl and pour into cauliflower mix, mix along with nutritional yeast, flour and corn meal.
4. Heat 1 tablespoons of coconut oil in the pan. Measure 1/4 cup of cauliflower mixture, pour into the pan and press the fritters down lightly to flatten.
5. Cook about 3 minutes per side or until all the fritters are golden brown.

Vanilla Chocolate Macaroon Bars

Prep time: 5 minutes
Cook time: 5 minutes
Servings: 12

Ingredients:
2 tsp of pure vanilla extract
Pinch of sea salt
1 tsp of cocoa powder or carob powder
1 tsp of ground cinnamon
2 cup of Medjool dates, pitted
2-4 tbsp of water
1/2 cup of almond butter
2 cup of raw almonds

Instructions:
1. Combine together all the ingredients one after another in a food processor, but reserve 2 tablespoon of water, pulse until mixture is smooth with a bit chunks of tiny almonds.
2. Forms mixture in a dough ball. Check the consistency and add more tablespoon of water if needed.
2. Place the dough on a cutting board and slice into 12 bars.
3. Wrapped and Store in the refrigerator.

Tasty Peach Crumble

Prep time: 5 minutes
Cook time: 35-45 minutes
Servings: 4-5

Ingredients:
1/8 cup of whole wheat flour
1 tablespoon of coconut oil
1 tablespoon of agave
1/2 teaspoon of ground cinnamon, divided
3/8 teaspoon of almond extract, alcohol-free
1 tablespoon of cornstarch
3 medium or 2 extra-large peaches, diced
3/8 cup of old-fashioned oats, possibly gluten-free

Instructions:
1. Heat up the oven to 350°F.
2. Toss diced peaches, 1/8 teaspoon of cinnamon, almond extract and cornstarch together in a medium bowl until fully combined.
3. Combine the remaining cinnamon, oats, and flour together in a separate bowl. Add in the coconut oil and 1 tablespoon agave, and keep mixing until totally incorporated.
4. In a 1 quart baking dish, spread the peach mixture, and sprinkle the oat flour crumbs evenly over the top.
5. Place the baking dish in the preheated oven and bake for 35-45 minute or until the oat mixture turns crunchy and peach juice starts to bubble. Let it completely cool. Best to allow it rest for 2 hours before serving after coming to room temperature so the juices can thicken.

Grilled Veggies With Tofu Skewers

Prep time: 20 minutes
Cook time: 10 minutes
Servings: 8

Ingredients:
2 tbsp of olive oil
4 tsps of chili powder
4 minced cloves garlic
10 tbsps. of fresh cilantro, chopped
1/4 tsps of cayenne pepper
Vegetables (thickly sliced zucchini, colorful bell peppers, red onion, summer/yellow squash and cherry tomatoes)
Salt and black pepper to taste
28 oz package firm tofu, drain as many water as possible
1/2 cup of fresh-squeezed lime juice

Instructions:
1. Arrange the tofu on a tray and cut horizontally, then into cubes.
2. Transfer the tofu pieces to a shallow dish.
3. Whisk together the chili powder, black pepper, olive oil, lime juice, cayenne pepper, garlic, cilantro (reserve 2 teaspoon) and salt together in a bowl.
4. Place the in the bowl and marinate in the marinade for 2-8 hours.
5. Pierce the tofu along with the veggies onto skewers.
6. Heat up an outdoor grill, and lightly grease the grate over medium heat.
7. Grill the pierced veggies and tofu, about 10 to 15 minutes, brushing occasionally with the marinade until almost blackened in spots.
8. To serve, sprinkle with fresh cilantro while still hot.

Made in the USA
Monee, IL
15 December 2021